INFRARED LIGHT THERAPY

For Recovery, Fitness, Skin Care, and Total-Body Wellness

MEDICAL DISCLAIMER

All content in this book is for informational purposes only.

This book is not intended to be a substitute for professional medical advice, diagnosis, or treatment. It is not intended to diagnose, treat, cure, or prevent any disease. Always seek the advice of your physician or other qualified health provider with any questions you may have regarding a medical condition. Never disregard professional medical advice or delay in seeking it because of something you have read in this book.

Copyright © 2021 Nancy Gordon Brooks & J.P. Roe

All rights reserved. No part of this book may be reproduced or used in any manner without permission of the copyright owner.

Table of Contents

Chapter One: What Is Light 1

Chapter Two: How Infrared Light Affects the Body 10

Chapter Three: Infrared Light Therapy 18

Chapter Four: Infrared Light Therapy Technology 33

Chapter Five: Infrared Light Therapy at Home 39

Chapter Six: Infrared Light Therapy Safety 46

Chapter Seven: Infrared Light Therapy FAQ 48

Glossary ii

Chapter One: What Is Light

Light is all around us and is an integral part of nearly every aspect of our lives. Among other things, it allows us to see, gives objects their colors, warms our bodies, and causes plants to grow. Sunlight is considered a requirement for both physical and emotional well-being. Electric light allows us to continue working and playing even after the sun has gone down.

While light itself is ubiquitous, an understanding of what makes up light and how it functions are not as common—at least outside of science and academia. Fortunately, the fundamentals of light can be explained without opening a single quantum physics textbook.

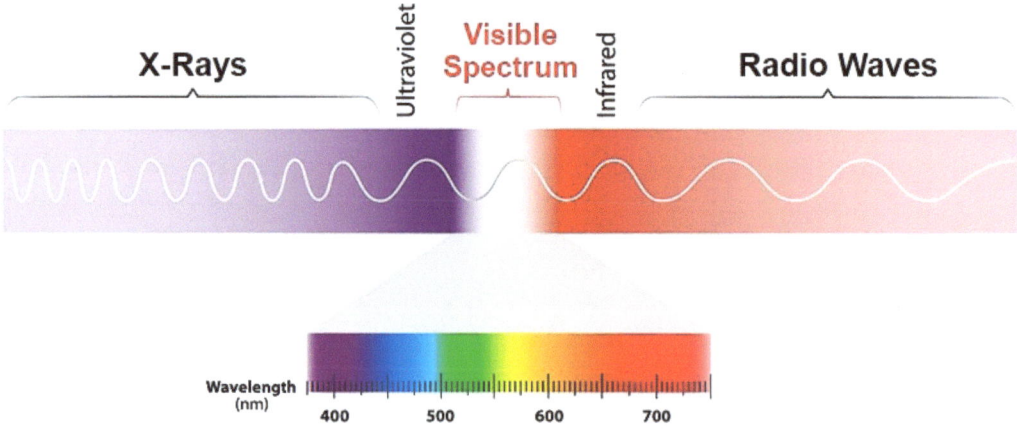

First, let's understand what light really is. Light is a type of electromagnetic energy, just like gamma rays, x-rays, microwaves, and radio signals. All of these types of energy are parts of the **electromagnetic spectrum,** which is a system of organizing these energy types for the purposes of study and discussion.

	Definition
electromagnetic spectrum	The range of radiation that encompasses gamma rays, x-rays, microwaves, and radio signals as well as visible and near infrared light.

Each type of energy travels in waves, which have troughs (lowest points) and peaks (highest points) just like waves on the ocean. What makes each type of energy different is the amount of time between the lowest to highest point. This amount of time is called **wavelength.**

wavelength	**Definition** A way of categorizing energy on the electromagnetic spectrum. The wavelength is the amount of time between the highest and lowest points on the wave of energy.

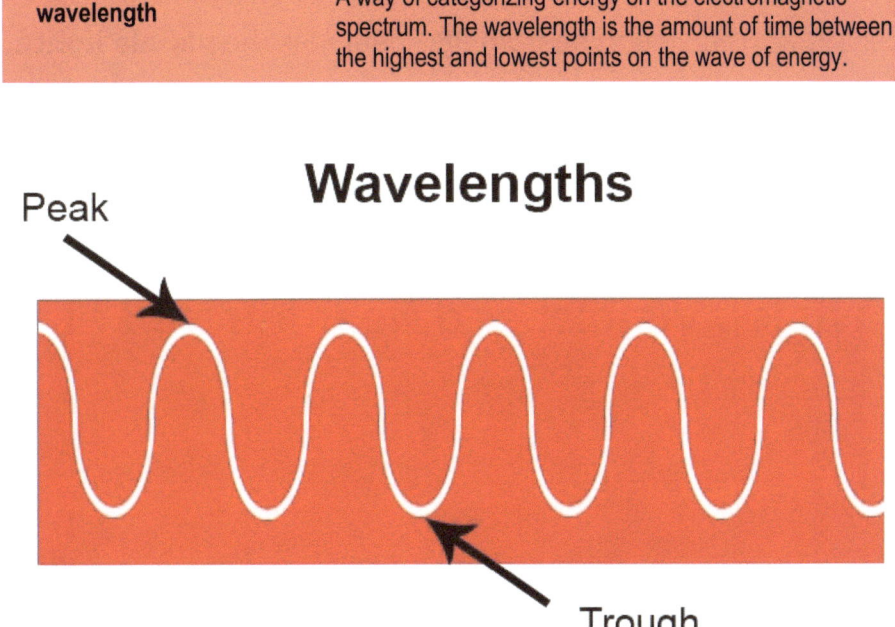

Energy that goes from trough to crest the fastest known is called short wavelength energy and those that go from lowest to highest point more slowly are called long wavelength energy. To even more precisely categorize these types of energy, scientists have assigned a unit of measure, called the **nanometer**(nm) to the wavelengths.

nanometer	**Definition** The unit of measure used to describe the wavelengths of the types of energy in the electromagnetic spectrum. It is abbreviated as nm.

Models of the electromagnetic spectrum arrange the various types of energy left to right, starting with the shortest wavelength:

- At the shortest wavelength end the light spectrum is **ultraviolet light**, which has wavelengths from 10nm-379nm.

- At the longest wavelength end is **infrared light**, which has wavelengths from 700nm-3000nm. It is further broken down into:
    - **near infrared light**, which is the wavelengths between 700nm-999nm)
    - **far infrared light**, which is the wavelengths between 1000nm and 3000nm)
- In the center, with wavelengths from 380-699nm is the **visible light** or **white light** spectrum. We can see these wavelengths and not others because the wavelengths comprising the visible spectrum stimulate the retina in the eye, turning the photons into nerve impulses in our brains.

Ultraviolet, Visible, and Near Infrared Light

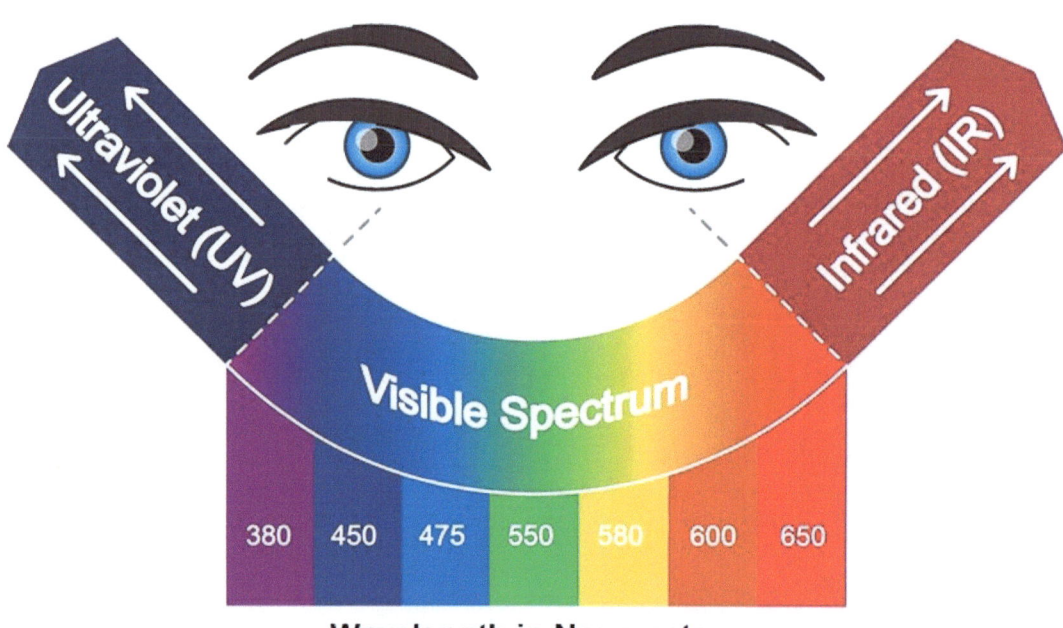

The visible light spectrum is further broken by the wavelengths that we see as different colors, ranging from violet to red. We can see this separation in nature, when the sun shines through raindrops and creates a rainbow.

Read More About . . .

Visible Light https://science.nasa.gov/ems/09_visiblelight

The Light Spectrum https://www.konicaminolta.com/instruments/knowledge/color/part2/02.html

What Can Light Do For Us?

Whether visible to the naked eye or not, light is constantly helping us in ways that are very familiar to us as well as some that we are just coming to understand. As we have discussed above, visible light is an integral part of everyday life. Infrared light from the sun keeps the earth warm. Ultraviolet (UV) light is absorbed by our skin and synthesized into Vitamin D, which is vital to the health of our teeth, bones, and muscles.

Medical researchers have, over the past few decades, been exploring other ways that light can help us. After all, we've proven that our body chemistry reacts to UV light in life-changing ways, so what other possibilities are out there? Eager for remedies and therapeutic benefits, these scientists have explored the use of various lasers and lamps in different wavelengths.

The results of such experiments, studies, and tests have been (pardon the pun) enlightening. We are now on the verge of a deeper understanding of the powerful impact light can have on our health and wellness.

Bioactive Light

Our bodies need certain types of light at certain times of the day to carry out many basic processes, including mood regulation, sleep and waking cycles, and cell repair. In fact, there are several well-known maladies are caused by a lack of light, including seasonal affective disorder (SAD) and rickets. Science is also uncovering negative effects that are caused by changes in the types of light we are exposed to and the times of day that we receive that exposure. These changes are the result of the use of new types of technology and changes in our ways of living.

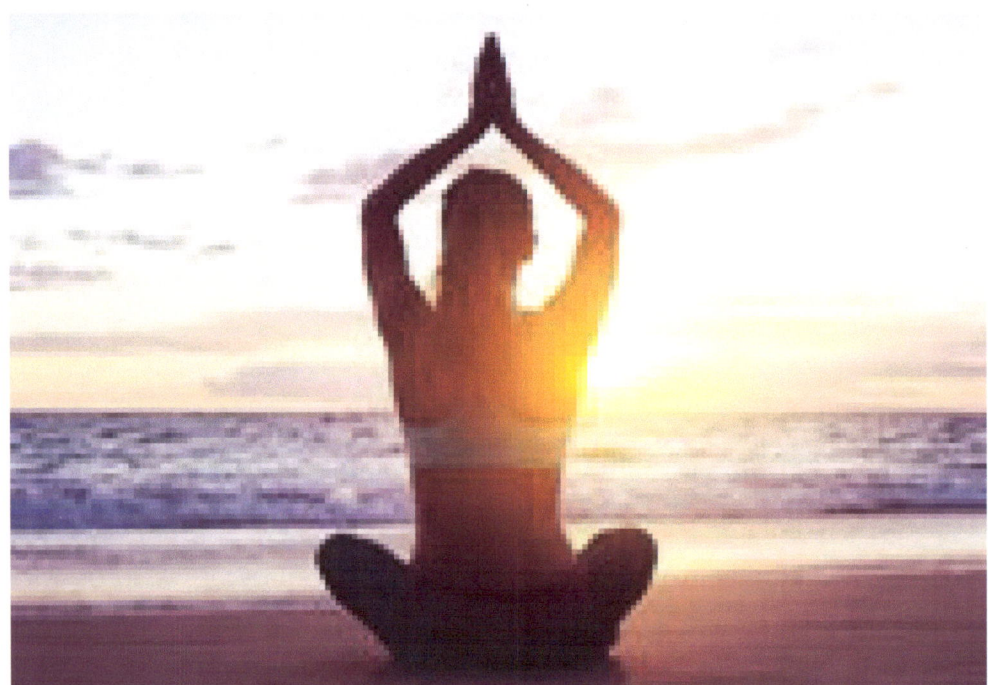

The types of light that are known to stimulate biological processes, including carry out vital functions and preventing maladies, are known as **bioactive light**.

| bioactive light | **Definition**
Forms of light that have some sort of measurable effect on the human body. These include UV light, Infrared light, and blue light. |

In the next few sections, we're going to examine four types of bioactive light and the changes they bring about in the human body:

- **UV Light** (10nm-379nm), which allows us to synthesize Vitamin D from sunlight

- **Blue Light** (380nm-449nm), which helps set and regulate our internal clocks

- **Red Light** (650-699nm) **and Near Infrared Light** (700nm-1000nm), which stimulate cellular energy production

- **Far Infrared Light** (1000nm-3000nm), which heats up our bodies and helps with circulation

UV Light

At the far end of the visible spectrum is a wavelength of light that's too short for us to see, called ultraviolet (UV) light or ultraviolet radiation. Sunlight is a natural source of UV light.

UV light is necessary for certain biological functions. For example, UV light helps our bodies synthesize the Vitamin D we need to maintain healthy bones and strengthens muscles and the immune system. It is also used in the treatment of certain skin conditions. Once such condition, psoriasis, causes the skin to shed cells too quickly and results in itchy, scaly patches.

Other research suggests that sunlight plays a key role in maintaining a healthy disposition. UV light from the sun stimulates the brain's pineal gland, causing it to produce a mood-enhancing chemical called tryptamine.

Blue Light

Right beside UV light on the spectrum, we find blue light. Blue light has a short wavelength with a high energy signature, which scatters more easily than other visible light. Computer screens, smartphones, and other digital devices that emit significant amounts of blue light can cause eye strain because of the high amount of unfocused, scattered light that they emit. Sunlight is also a source of blue light.

Blue Light

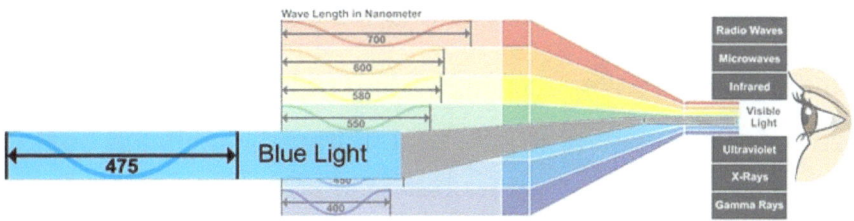

While blue wavelengths are beneficial during daylight hours because they boost attention, reaction times, and mood, they become disruptive at night. Blue light exposure near bedtime can throw off our circadian rhythms. It has also been shown to cause sleep disruption by significantly reducing production of the hormone melatonin during sleep.

Scientists are linking increases in several modern health issues, including diabetes and obesity, to our heightened exposure to blue light from technology such as computer screens, smart phones, and LED televisions.

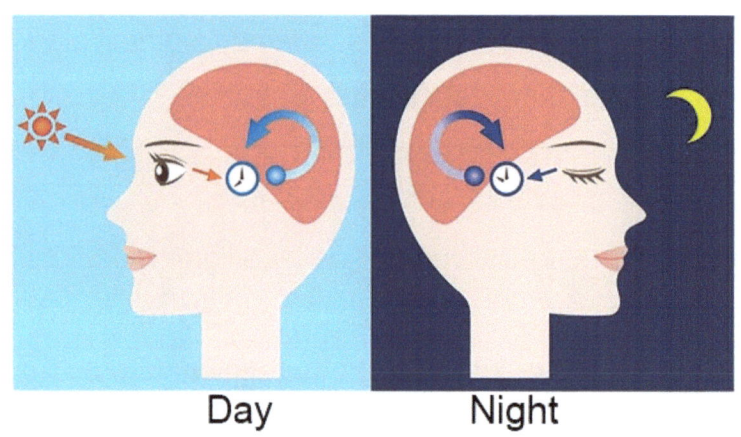

Read More About . . .

Potential Health Effects of Blue Light https://www.health.harvard.edu/staying-healthy/blue-light-has-a-dark-side

Red and Infrared Light

At the far end of the visible light spectrum, we find red light. Immediately next to red light is closely-related but invisible infrared (IR) light. Infrared light is the heat you feel from sunlight and radiating from a camp fire or hot sidewalk. Your skin naturally puts out infrared heat as a byproduct of biological functioning.

Infrared light helps our bodies perform multiple important functions. It aids in cell repair and regeneration. It can increase blood circulation, which has been shown to promote collagen production, faster healing and reduce symptoms of chronic pain.

Infrared light can penetrate below the skin layers, typically two to seven centimeters below the surface, reaching muscles, nerves, and even bone. Once inside the body, infrared light is absorbed by the photoreceptors in cells. The light energy sets off a series of metabolic events, which trigger several natural cellular processes.

Red and Near Infrared Light Penetration

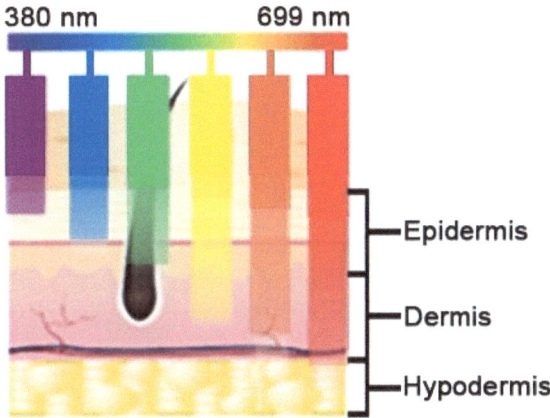

One of these processes is the production of nitric oxide production. **Nitric oxide**, a gas that's vital to the health of the circulatory system, is a cellular signaling molecule that helps relax the arteries, reduce oxidative stress, prevent clotting in the vessels, and regulate blood pressure. In doing so, nitric oxide enhances circulation to deliver vital nutrients and oxygen-rich blood to damaged tissues in the body. This stimulates the regeneration and repair at injury sites, reducing pain and inflammation.

	Definition
nitric oxide	A chemical that is comprised of a nitrogen atom and an oxygen atom. It performs a number of activities in the body relative to cellular function.

Read More About . . .

Oxidative Stress https://www.healthline.com/health/oxidative-stress

Potential Benefits of Red Light Therapy https://www.healthline.com/health-news/red-light-therapy-benefits

Anti-inflammatory effects of Red and Near Infrared Light www.aimspress.com/article/10.3934/biophy.2017.3.337/fulltext.html

Red and Near Infrared Light and Muscle Tissue https://onlinelibrary.wiley.com/doi/abs/10.1002/jbio.201600176

Chapter Two: How Infrared Light Affects the Body

Now that we have a general understanding of light and some of its effects on the body, we are going to take a detailed look at one particular type of bioactive light: infrared light. In so doing we're going to provide information that will help you understand whether or not infrared light therapy is right for you.

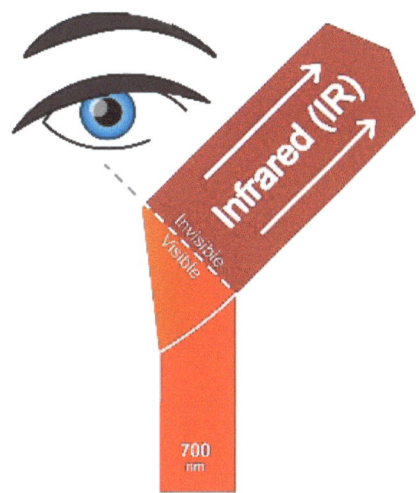

Specifically, we're going to get answers to the following questions:

- What does infrared do to the skin?
- How does infrared light promote healing?
- How can invisible light help with pain?

Please keep in mind that this information is not intended to be medical advice and that you should always consult with a medical professional before beginning any sort of therapeutic regimen, including infrared light therapy.

Stimulating ATP

When researching infrared light, you'll see the term **photobiomodulation** come up quite a bit. This is because red light therapy is designed to enhance cellular function and promote greater efficiency and balance in the cellular energy-making process. Which is, in a nutshell, what's happening during photobiomodulation.

	Definition
photobiomodulation	Using red and near infrared light to trigger chemical changes within cells.

Let's go all the way back to basic biology. We each have trillions of cells in our bodies, and each one needs energy to function. This energy comes from the food, water, and oxygen that we bring into our bodies and metabolize through the process of **cellular respiration**.

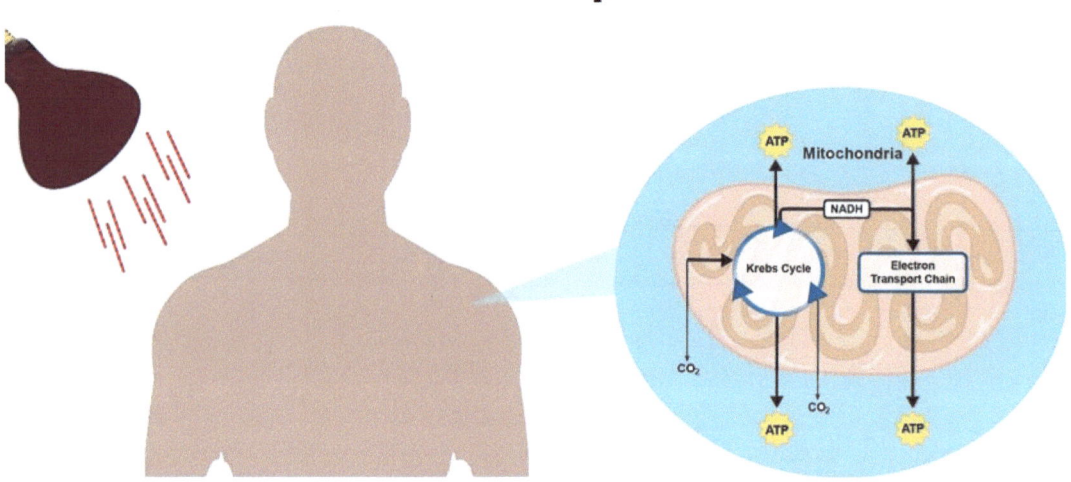

	Definition
cellular respiration	The process carried out by cells to convert fuel to energy and nutrients.

The product of cellular respiration is **adenosine triphosphate (ATP)**, a carrier of energy that our body is both constantly producing and consuming. The more efficiently we can create ATP, the better we feel and function.

	Definition
adenosine triphosphate	A molecule that carries energies within a cell; often referred to as a cell's "power plant."

Infrared light makes the cellular respiration process more efficient and, in turn, helps your body make and use ATP energy more effectively. Infrared light exerts its influence directly on the mitochondria, the powerhouses of the cell. Red light therapy can both increase the number of mitochondria and boost their efficiency.

This boost comes from stimulating the electrons of the mitochondria during cellular respiration, helping to clear out nitric oxide, which is, a barrier to ATP production. Nitric oxide can build up almost like sludge in a car's engine and, like that sludge, it can make it harder for normal processes—in this case ATP production—to be carried out.

IR light, along with red light, flush out nitric oxide to help prevent and reverse this problem. The photons in these types of light are temporarily absorbed by the electrons in the nitric oxide molecule, which is known as exciting the electrons. In this state, the bonds in the molecule break down, which allows hydrogen ions to move through the cellular respiration process more easily.

Infrared Light's Effect on Nitric Oxide

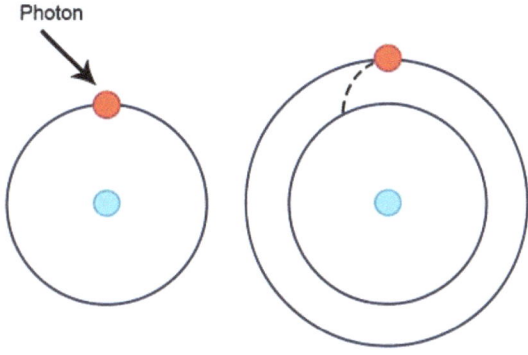

Read More About . . .

Atoms and Light Energy https://go.nasa.gov/3qrbxZxt

Now we'll take a closer look at each step of this process.

The Mitochondria in Cells Power the Body

Mitochondria are double-membrane structures in our cells responsible for a number of processes, including cell signaling, steroid synthesis, and cellular energy. Mitochondria are unique, with their own ribosomes and DNA. There can be as few as 1-2 mitochondria per cell, or as many as thousands.

The number of mitochondria changes in response to such conditions such as exercise, nutrients, and certain environmental factors.

Mitochondria

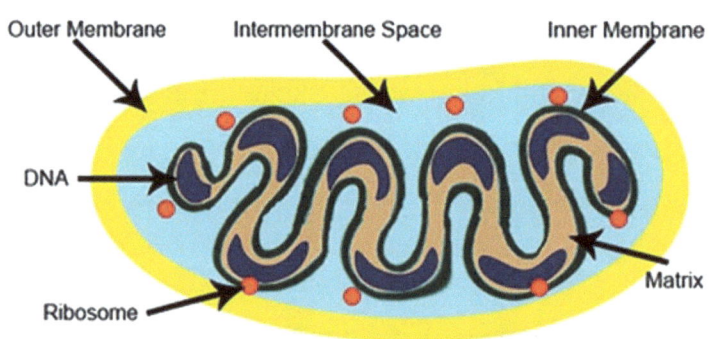

What is Adenosine Triphosphate (ATP)?

As we mentioned earlier, mitochondria convert food, water, and oxygen into ATP energy that the cells and body can use. In fact, the average person recycles an amount of ATP equal to his or her own body weight every day. ATP energy fuels everything we do. It is so critical for biological function, it's often called "the energy currency of life." Therefore, the more efficiently cells can make and use ATP energy, the better the body should function.

This is where red and near infrared light enter the picture. These types of light energy can help enhance both the number of mitochondria in a cell and the ability of the mitochondria to make ATP.

Infrared Light Science

Infrared light improves mitochondrial function by removing a barrier to ATP production. It breaks the chemical bonds between nitric oxide and a substance called cytochrome C oxidase (Cox) that is a critical part of cellular respiration. When nitric oxide binds to Cox, it occupies space that should be taken up by oxygen. Less oxygen in the mitochondria makes the cell work less efficiently, which reduces the production of ATP.

The presence of nitric oxide also increases the number of free radical molecules, which are oxygen molecules with uneven numbers of electrons. This uneven number causes these molecules to seek out other molecules and bind to them, which can often result in reactions that are harmful to the body. You have likely heard foods and cosmetics advertised as being or containing anti-oxidants. These substances also have uneven numbers of electrons and are introduced to the body to bind to the free radicals so that they are no longer able to do damage.

Red and near infrared light reduce the harm that nitric oxide can do. Their photons excite the electrons in the nitric oxide, which break the bonds with Cox, freeing up space for oxygen and allowing hydrogen atoms to move free, which result in increased production of ATP.

Read More About . . .

Mitochondria	https://www.cell.com/current-biology/fulltext/S0960-9822(06)01781-7
How Does Infrared Therapy Work?	https://bit.ly/3vVglKn

Therapeutic Heat

Treating the body using high or low temperatures, or thermotherapy, is designed to alter tissue temperature over time to induce a desirable biological response. Heating pads, hot water bottles, heated blankets, and ice packs are all familiar home remedies used for thermotherapy. They deliver a temperature change to a specific area of the body without affecting much of the surrounding tissue.

As you probably know, cold (ice packs, cold compresses) is usually used on burns or immediately after tissue injuries to reduce swelling. On the other hand, heat is primarily used for relaxation, comfort, and exercise recovery. Heat also can reduce several kinds of discomfort, such as dull and persistent pains associated with stiffness, cramping, and strains. More specifically, heat is often applied in these general pain and soreness situations:

- Acute soreness from overexertion and exercise.
- Stiffness and pain in specific areas related to arthritis, muscle knots, and most kinds of cramps.
- General pain and sensitivity from afflictions such as fibromyalgia, arthritis, drug side effects, Vitamin D deficiency, and sleep deprivation.

Effect of Heat on Bloodflow

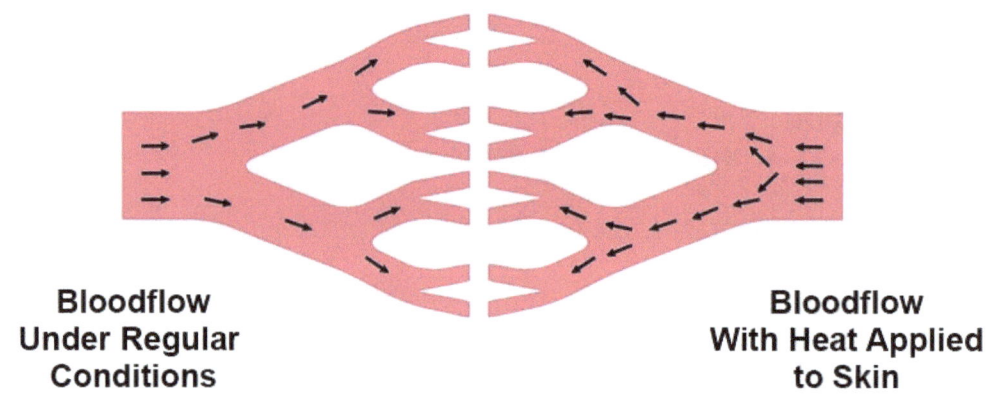

Bloodflow Under Regular Conditions

Bloodflow With Heat Applied to Skin

Deep heating is thought to:

Decrease:

▶ nerve sensitivity

▶ muscle spindle sensitivity to stretch

Increase:

▶ muscle relaxation

▶ tissue metabolism (via photobiomodulation)

▶ flexibility

▶ blood flow

One of the well-documented benefits of heat therapy, including the deep penetrating heat from infrared light, is improved blood flow. Heat stimulates receptors that are connected to the blood vessels in the skin, which causes the release of a substance that relaxes the walls of the blood vessels, allowing them to become larger and more blood to pass through them. Blood flow directly impacts healing and inflammation. Since inflammation is a component of many types of pain, the simple application of heat can work wonders.

Read More About . . .

Thermotherapy   https://www.physio-pedia.com/Thermotherapy

Effects of Infrared Light on Skin

With skin being the largest organ in your body, skin care is not just about beauty (although that's important, too). Your skin plays a vital role in immunity, body temperature, and hormone regulation. The myriad of important functions of the skin are

Collagen and Aging

the result of millions of cells working together and communicating with one another. When the mitochondria in those skin cells absorb healthy red and NIR light, they not only produce more energy (ATP), but more pro-collagen, collagen, basic fibroblast growth factors (bFGF), and fibroblasts. These components are critical to maintaining skin elasticity and overall health. Collagen alone makes up approximately 75% of skin's support structure. Collagen production decreases with age and is also damaged by free radicals and environmental factors, such as too much sunlight and smoking. Through its heat-therapy powers of vasodilation, red light therapy can also increase microcirculation, which improves cellular balance.

All of these benefits work together to promote healthy balance. Balanced skin cells operating at full capacity do all of their jobs better, giving you healthier, glowing skin that looks and feels fantastic.

Chapter Three: Infrared Light Therapy

Infrared light can be used for a variety of beneficial purposes, including pain relief and improvement in skin tone and appearance. In this chapter we'll look at some of the therapeutic uses for near infrared and red light therapies, examine the science behind them, and discuss studies that have been used to evaluate their effectiveness.

Research Into NIR and Pain

A number of studies that have documented the effectiveness of infrared light in relieving indicators of pain from multiple causes and in multiple locations on the body. These include chronic and acute pain, pain from injuries and pain from overexertion. In one of them, a Rothbart Pain Management Clinic study, infrared energy was delivered to 40 people who suffered from chronic lower back pain. The method was shown to be effective in reducing chronic lower back pain with zero adverse side effects.

Read More About . . .

Infrared Therapy for Chronic Low Back Pain   https://www.ncbi.nlm.nih.gov/pmc/articles/PMC2539004/

Another study, published in the Turkish Journal of Physical Medicine and Rehabilitation, looked at the impact of infrared light therapy on inflammatory arthritis of the spine. In the study, patients treated with infrared light experienced improved mobility, function, and quality of life.

Read More About . . .

Light Therapy for Arthritis of the Spine   https://bit.ly/2P2OyqP

In light therapy (infrared light therapy, red light therapy, dual optical energy, low light laser therapy, and others), certain wavelengths of bioreactive light energy are delivered to sites of the body where there is pain or injury. Near infrared (NIR) light therapy specifically uses wavelengths between 700nm and 1000nm.

How Infrared Light Therapy Works

NIR therapy has been shown to have direct effects on pain signaling pathways. Studies of the effectiveness of light therapy on a number of chronic pain conditions suggest that it may affect nerve fibers involved in conduction of pain signals. Human and animal studies have found elevated levels of **endorphins** (small proteins that block pain signals in nerves) in response to light therapy, as well as several other biochemical effects that can produce a net benefit in terms of pain relief.

Infrared light also stimulates the flow of nitric oxide. Nitric oxide occurs naturally in the body and is a signaling molecule which plays a major role in promoting blood flow to tissues. Increased blood flow helps bring oxygen and nutrients to injured areas. Infrared light also enhances lymphatic drainage, which means that inflammation is inhibited and swelling is reduced.

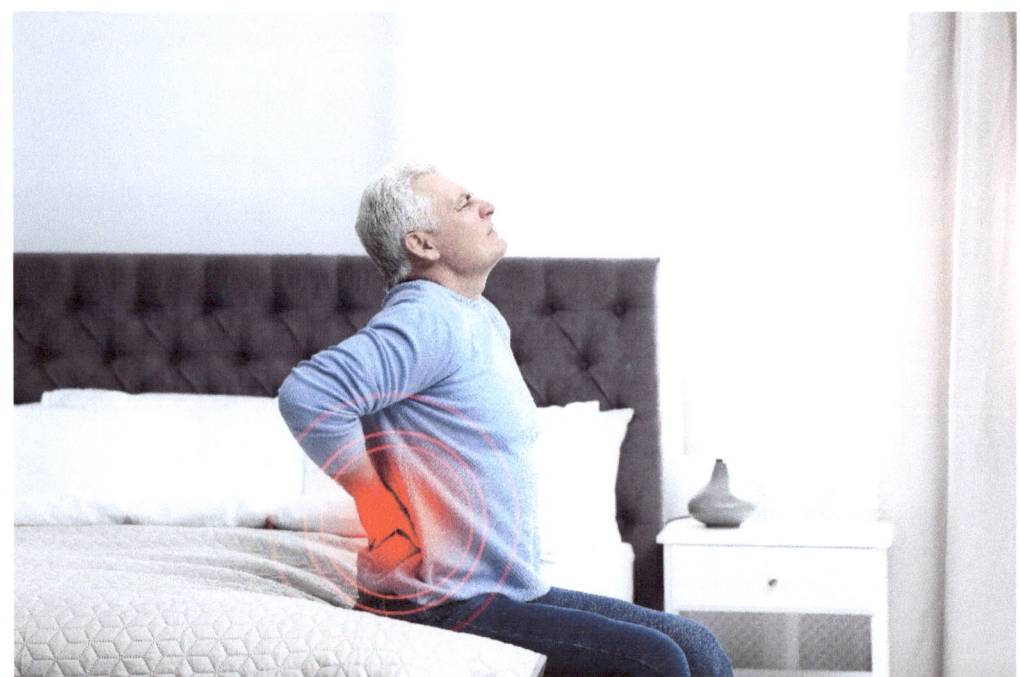

All this means that infrared light therapy can treat pain indicators from deep muscle tissue, bones, and joints. It can also help with associated problems like swelling. Since infrared light penetrates deep into the skin, muscle tissue, and even bone, it is able to deliver potential benefits throughout most of the body.

Pain Relief

Pain management is an integral part of health care. It can also be subject of intense disagreement. Healthcare practitioners and lawmakers are challenged to provide effective pain relief while ensuring that patients do not become dependent upon the medication prescribed to them. Heavy monitoring, restrictions, and a desire to avoid addiction and other side effects have patients looking for alternatives to pharmaceutical pain management. Everything from acupuncture to essential oils, to herbal supplements are being touted as natural pain relievers.

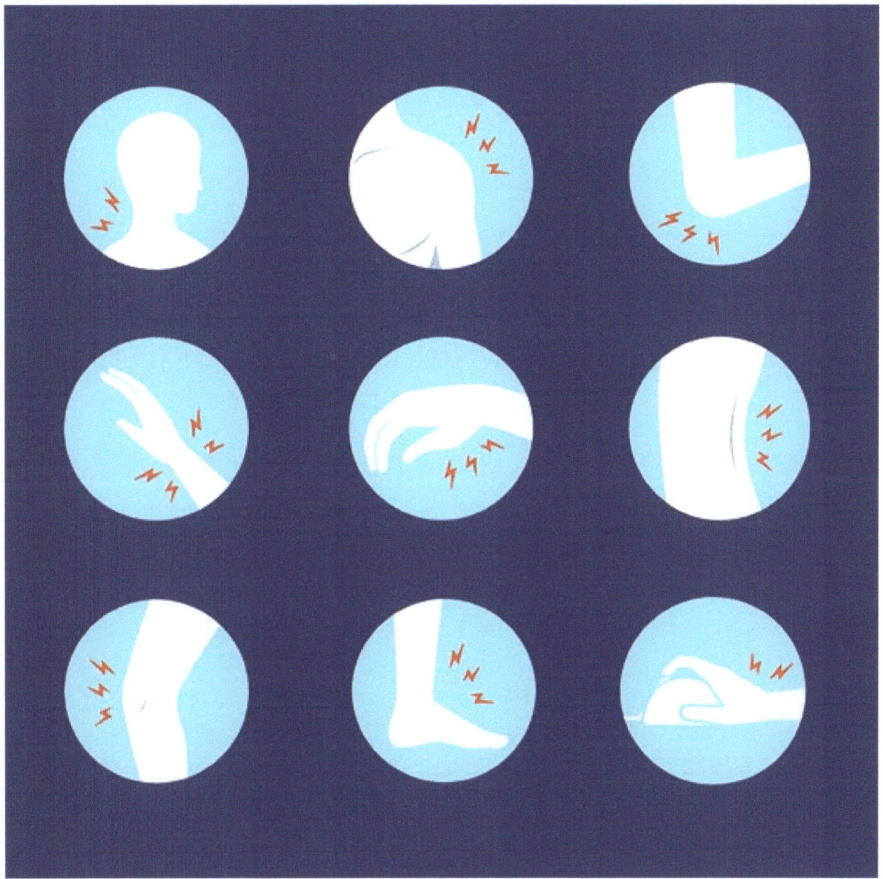

And then there's infrared light therapy. Perhaps the most non-invasive means of addressing both chronic and acute pains in current use, infrared and red light therapy truly "shed new light" on the issue of safe, legal pain relief.

What Types of Pain Can Infrared Light Therapy Treat?

Infrared light therapy can treat chronic and temporary inflammation, making it useful in the treatment of:

- Osteoarthritis and rheumatoid arthritis
- Chronic neck pain
- Chronic back pain
- Tendon Inflammation
- Sore muscles and joints from exercise or rehabilitative therapy
- Diabetic neuropathy
- Foot and ankle pain
- Hands, when tired and achy from arthritis or other issues
- Sciatica
- Neck aches and stiffness
- Shoulder soreness
- Wounds and post-surgical incisions
- Carpal tunnel syndrome
- Upper back pain

Read More About . . .

NIR for Peripheral Neuropathy	https://clinicaltrials.gov/ct2/show/NCT00125268
Photobiomodulation in Clinical Trials	https://pubmed.ncbi.nlm.nih.gov/28547075/
Near Infrared and Muscle Soreness	https://pubmed.ncbi.nlm.nih.gov/16538423/
Near Infrared and Skeletal Muscle Inflammation	https://pubmed.ncbi.nlm.nih.gov/25200395/

Why Choose Infrared Light Therapy Over Other Home Options?

There was a time when infrared therapy was an expensive option that involved specialized equipment available only in clinical settings. This is no longer the case.

Infrared light bulbs designed for home use are widely available. These bulbs require no special equipment to operate and screw into a standard light socket. You can use the bulbs in high wattage clamp lamp from the hardware store or combine several clamp lamps and bulbs and turn an unused closet into your own infrared sauna for less than $200.

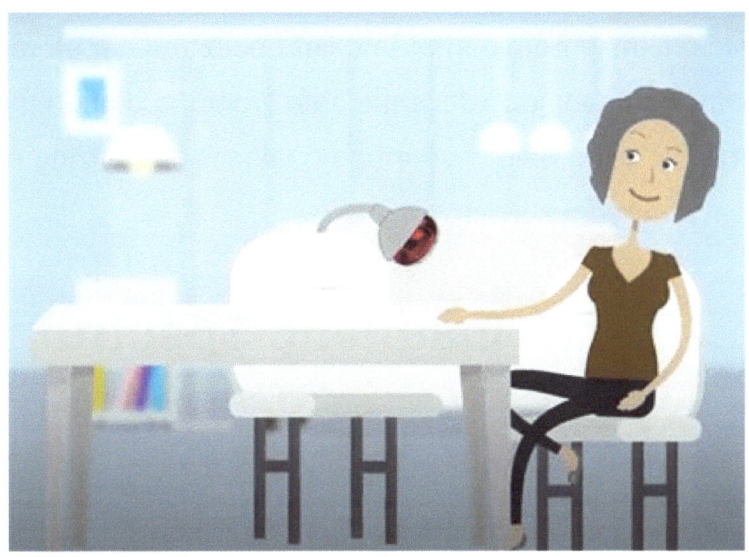

Even though NIR therapy has become simpler and more cost-effective, you may be wondering what advantages infrared light offer over other home therapy options.

First off, there is an extensive amount of evidence, including formal research studies, that support its efficacy. You can choose to try this approach without worrying that it's a gimmick or "snake oil". There's even plenty of testimonials and case studies from real users just like you to support the research.

Not only is infrared light therapy affordable to start with, but it involves very little recurring cost. Unlike supplements, creams, teas, or medications that get used up, your NIR bulb can be used over and over again for many months or years. Once you've made the initial purchase, you can enjoy relief day after day without having to refill a prescription or restock your supply.

Lastly, home infrared light therapy is safe, so long as you purchase bulbs that are free from toxic substances and, if you are sensitive to EMF, you choose incandescent bulbs. Incandescent bulbs are designed to operate in a manner that does not produce EMF.

Is Infrared Energy Dangerous?

Do infrared therapy lamps emit radiation? Technically, yes, all energy on the electromagnetic spectrum is radiation. Radiation simply refers to the output of energy, which can apply to anything from a standard light bulb to a car stereo. Infrared light energy is non-ionizing, meaning that it's the safe type of radiation that doesn't have enough energy to alter molecules in your body. Other non-ionizing radiation sources include visible light and radio waves.

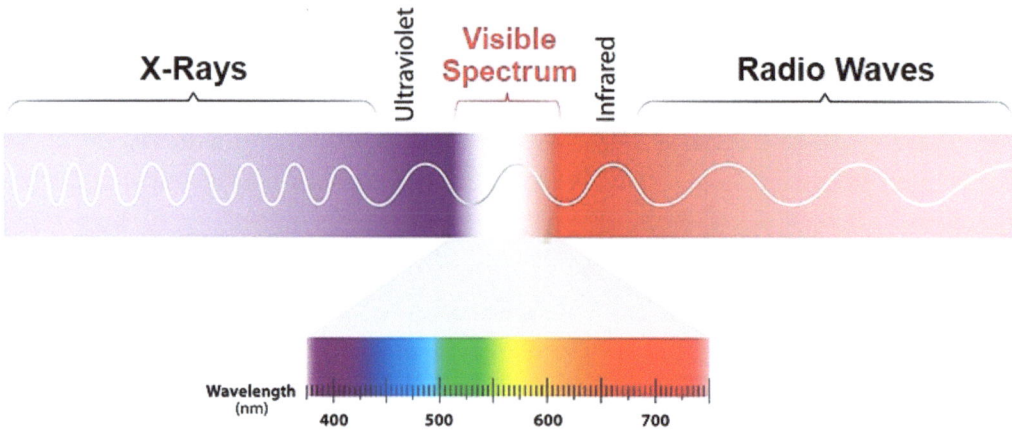

Red and infrared light therapy that uses traditional **incandescent** lightbulbs involves heat (some higher-wattage bulbs reach nearly 600° Fahrenheit), so you will want to be mindful of this when using the bulb and maintain a comfortable distance. You'll also want to take the same safety measures that you would with any electrical device that produces heat.

incandescent lightbulb	**Definition** A bulb that produces light and heat as a result of electrical current passing through a metal filament.

How Can I Get the Safest and Most Effective Therapy Products?

As we mentioned, your overall experience with infrared light therapy can hinge on the quality of your equipment, as well as your knowledge going in. To get the most out of your therapy, it's wise to use the best infrared therapy bulbs and set them up according to the information found in Chapter Six.

Always choose a bulb that is designed to maximize red and near infrared output. Bulbs that are marketed as full spectrum bulbs emit primarily visible, and sometimes UV light, but produce little to no near infrared light. Many general purpose heat lamp bulbs, such as those sold at hardware stores, are designed primarily to produce heat and are used for everything from warming an entryway to heating food on a buffet line.

These bulbs also produce red and near infrared light, but are not designed specifically to emit these wavelengths, nor are they manufactured with the understanding that people will be using them on the human body, for therapeutic purposes.

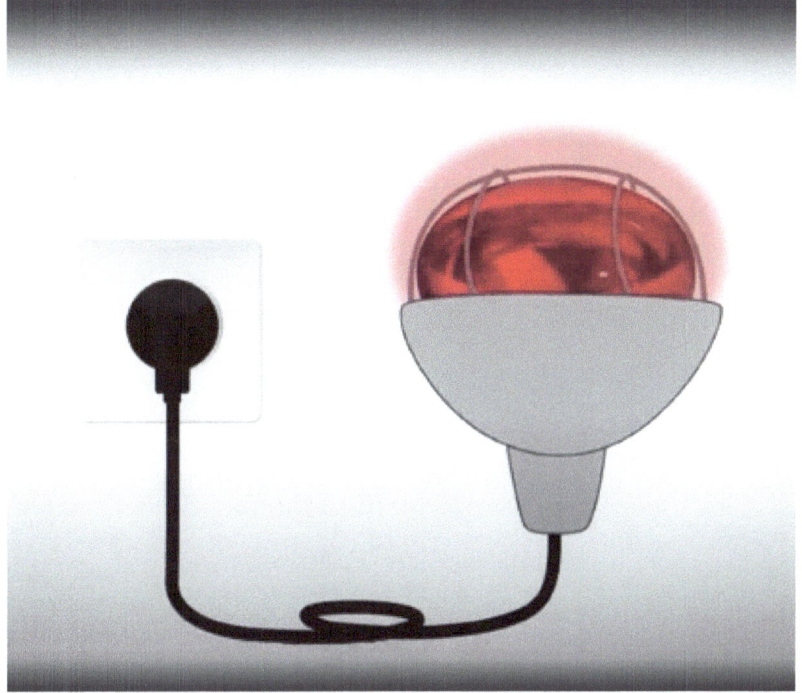

An effective product is one that is accompanied by information on:

- Total wavelength range
- Percentage of output by wavelength
- Peak wavelength
- Intensity, also known as irradiance

This information should be lab-verified, especially because near infrared energy is invisible to the naked eye. Without a third-party verification, you have no way of knowing for sure if the bulb puts out any NIR energy.

In addition to verifying what comes out the bulbs, you will want to know what goes into them to make sure that you are not exposing yourself to such hazardous substances as Teflon, mercury, and lead. A bulb that bears an RoHS (Restriction of Hazardous Substances Directive) certification offers the assurance that it is free of these and other hazardous materials. An additional certification, known as a CE Marking, indicates that the bulb has been manufactured to European Economic Area (EEA) standards for health, safety, and environmental protection.

Read More About . . .

RoHS https://www.rohsguide.com/

CE Marking http://www.ce-marking.org/what-is-ce-marking.html

Be sure to pair them with a lamp that's rated to operate bulbs with wattage at or above the wattage of the bulb. If you are choosing a bulb that is 250W or 300W, we recommend a lamp that has a ceramic socket. Clamp lamps that are rated at 300W are available at your nearest hardware store or online and will work well for this purpose.

NIR Therapy for Lyme Disease

Lyme Disease is the most common tick-borne illness in North America. More than 30,000 cases of Lyme Disease are reported in the U.S. every year, but that is only a small percentage of the actual number of cases. The Centers for Disease Control (CDC), estimates that up to 300,000 Americans get Lyme disease each year.

As you may already know, Lyme disease is transmitted to humans through infected blacklegged ticks. It is most commonly reported in the Northeastern US, where these ticks are abundant and active, but has been reported throughout the US and even in the UK. Symptoms include fever, headache, fatigue, and a characteristic "bullseye"-shaped skin rash. If left untreated, Lyme Disease infection can spread to joints, the heart, and the nervous system. [Hu LT. Lyme Disease. Ann Intern Med. 2016 Nov 1;165(9):677.]

The typical treatment for Lyme disease is antibiotics. Antibiotic use often is accompanied by unpleasant side effects. However, studies have shown that infrared sauna therapy can be used with antibiotics to speed healing. As we've discussed in the previous chapter, infrared energy has the ability to penetrate deep below the skin's surface. This can have a detoxifying effect, which is one of the primary objectives in treating Lyme disease.

Many of those living with Lyme disease often report joint pain in their shoulder or lower back. Anecdotally, they have reported relief from IR therapy via a single bulb or an IR sauna. Infrared heat's ability to increase blood circulation by penetrating deeper into the body's joints, muscles and tissues allows more oxygen to reach injured areas of the body and reduces inflammation, helping to reduce pain associated with Lyme disease.

Skin Care

Taking care of your skin is vital not only for your appearance, but for your overall health Skin plays a huge role in everything from immunity, to body temperature regulation, to hormone balance. Near infrared and red light therapy treatments can enhance cellular function and promote healthier skin across your entire body.

What Impact Does Skin Health Have on Overall Health?

Our skin is the largest organ we have, and it's the first line of defense for our immune system. Skin plays a key role in other bodily processes as well, including blood circulation, hormone production, and temperature regulation. Here's a look at some of the most important things our skin does for us:

- **Protection and Immunity:** The skin is our barrier against the world, from dirt and debris as well as germs and diseases. Skin is an essential component of a healthy immune system, fighting off dangers ranging from radiation to infections.

- **Circulation and Repair:** Blood flow brings oxygen and nutrients to the skin while at the same time carrying away carbon dioxide and waste products.

- **Storage and Hormone Production:** The deeper layers of our skin are storerooms for such critical substances as water, fat, and metabolic products. Our skin also produces key hormones such as Vitamin D, which is made with exposure to sunlight.

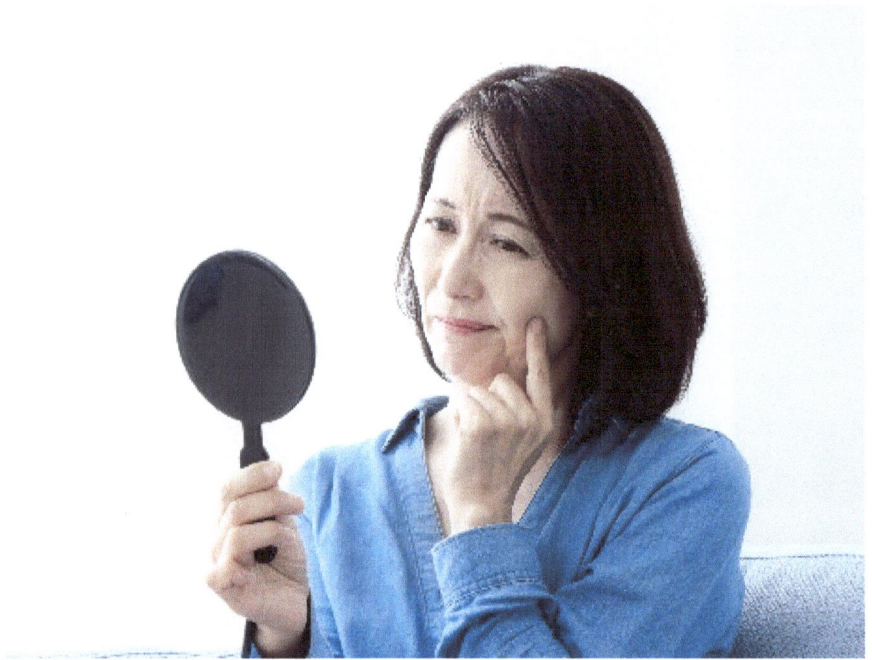

- **Temperature Regulation:** The skin is essential to body temperature regulation, protecting you from heat or cold, and helping to prevent dehydration.
- **Beauty:** Your skin plays a much larger role than just appearance, but that doesn't mean appearance isn't important too. Skin is central to how we perceive ourselves, and how others view us, which affects self-esteem and day-to-day mental health.

Red and Near Infrared Therapy and Skin Health

NIR/red light therapy, also known as photobiomodulation, is a simple, non-invasive treatment that delivers wavelengths of red and near infrared (NIR) light to the skin and cells. Red light therapy works by enhancing cellular function. Wavelengths of red and NIR light have been shown to stimulate the mitochondria, the powerhouse of the cell, and can optimize the cellular respiration process that makes ATP (adenosine triphosphate) energy. These treatments are quick and easy and expose the user to red and NIR light. Want to dive deeper into how this works at the cellular level?

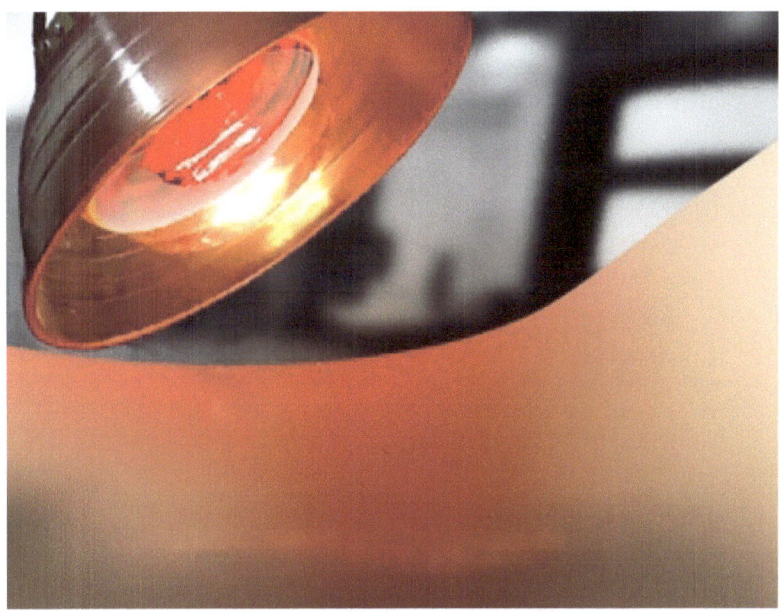

Taking in light is crucial for skin health, and overall health and wellness. Our bodies work better, and even look better, when our cells are in a state of balance, or homeostasis. Red and NIR light promote balance across the body by enhancing the cellular environment, making energy production more efficient, and decreasing inflammation and oxidative stress. When your cells are in greater balance, your skin will look and feel softer and more invigorated.

How NIR and Red Light Support Skin Health

NIR/red light therapy can help support skin health across the entire body. The skin functions mentioned above all rely on millions of cells performing and communicating with one another. When the mitochondria in those skin cells absorb healthy red and NIR light, they can produce more energy (ATP), stimulating the synthesis of pro-collagen, collagen, basic fibroblast growth factors (bFGF), and proliferation of fibroblasts. Red light therapy can also increase microcirculation, which improves cellular balance. In summary, balanced skin cells operating at full capacity do all of these jobs better. That can translate to healthier, glowing skin that looks and feels smoother and softer.

Inflammation can wreak havoc on skin health and appearance. In addition to supporting cellular health, NIR/red light therapy, combined with a healthy lifestyle, has been shown to have a positive impact on inflammation. Dr. Michael Hamblin of Harvard Medical School is a leading light therapy researcher. Dr. Hamblin has written about how NIR/red light therapy has the potential to reduce oxidative stress and increase blood flow to damaged and inflamed tissues. This can help skin tissue regenerate and heal faster, reducing inflammation and improving bodily balance.

Basic Fibroblast Growth Factors

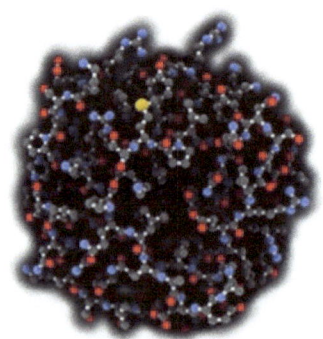

Why Use Red Light Therapy for Full-Body Skin Health?

Years ago, near infrared and red light therapy was almost exclusive to high-end salons and spas that used them for skin treatments. Thanks to innovations in bulb technology, this therapy is now accessible to just about anyone. Aestheticians and home users have taken notice and many of the world's leading skin experts have made infrared and red light therapy a part of their skincare routines.

While your face tends to get the most attention when you're planning a care regimen, healthy skin is a whole-body idea. NIR treatments make it easy to take your entire body into account. The more of your skin you can expose to healthy wavelengths of light, the more cellular activity is increased, which translates to better overall health. True health and beauty are often best attained through a full-body approach.

Supporting Skin Health with Infrared and Red Light Therapy

Vibrant, healthy skin is essential for your well-being as a whole. Healthy skin is vital for immunity, circulation, hormone balance, and temperature regulation. It's important to take care of more than just your face, and getting healthy light from head to toe, while maintaining a balanced lifestyle is an important step.

Infrared Saunas (Whole Body Care)

An infrared sauna is an enclosure that contains a source of near infrared energy and heat. It is designed to detoxify and heal the body, boost mood, and provide other benefits. Unlike traditional saunas that feature steam to warm the space, infrared saunas use infrared bulbs in confined spaces to raise body temperature directly.

Because infrared heat penetrates human tissue versus simply heating skin, infrared saunas promote circulation throughout the body, which can lead to increased metabolism, muscle and joint pain relief, boosted immune system, and, of course, stress and fatigue reduction.

Infrared heat is very gentle and essentially mimics the effects of lying in the sun on a warm day without the dangers of UV light. Unlike traditional hot rock or steam saunas, infrared saunas offer the benefit of being effective at a more comfortable operating temperature. Additionally, an infrared sauna requires no special cabinet, electrical hookup, or expensive specialized equipment. They're fast becoming the easiest and most accessible way to achieve that fresh-from-the-spa glow, even at home.

Read More About . . .

Clinical Effects of Infrared Sauna Use https://www.ncbi.nlm.nih.gov/pmc/articles/PMC5941775/

Near Infrared and Bone Repair

Bone density and the ability of the body to regrow bones is important for those recovering from injuries. Time is also a factor, as our bones tend to become increasingly brittle with age, in turn increasing our risk of fractures. Studies have documented positive results in the use of infrared and red light to promote bone health, especially for the treatment and healing of bone injuries, and the reduction of pain and swelling around injury sites.

Research has shown that near infrared and red light can have the following positive effects on bone health:

- Facilitates bone healing
- Improves bone structure and density
- Increases natural collagen production
- Improve bone biomechanical properties and overall strength

Fracture Repair

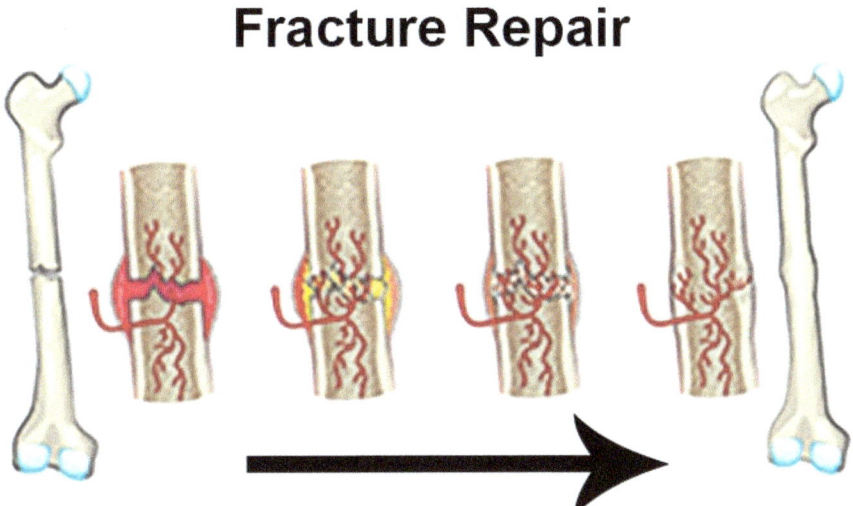

Red and near infrared light wavelengths are able to penetrate deep into tissue and bone to deliver their healing effects. Concentrated bioactive light stimulates the mitochondria at the cellular level to reduce oxidative stress and help the body to produce more usable energy. This energy is then used to fuel regenerative and healing processes.

Chapter Four: Infrared Light Therapy Technology

NIR light is often grouped under the broader umbrella of red light therapy, as well as low-level laser therapy or photobiomodulation. This is technically incorrect, as each of these techniques use different parts of the light spectrum. Red light uses rays with wavelengths ranging from 650nm-699nm and NIR ranges from 700nm-1000nm. To further complicate matters, the terms "near infrared" and "infrared" are often used interchangeably, but are not synonymous. Infrared refers to all energy with wavelengths between 700nm and 3000nm. Near infrared is a subset of this spectrum, with wavelengths from 700nm – 1000nm.

NIR therapy devices produce calibrated wavelengths of light in concentrations that provide therapeutic benefits at the cellular level without the dangers of excessive heat. To deliver the desired results, NIR therapy devices must produce a strong and focused beam of light that's capable of penetrating into the site. The therapy light needs a direct path to the skin and enough energy to make it through the skin and muscle tissue. There are a number of technologies that have these properties. In the remainder of this chapter, we will look at two devices that are designed and priced for home use.

Incandescent Infrared Bulbs

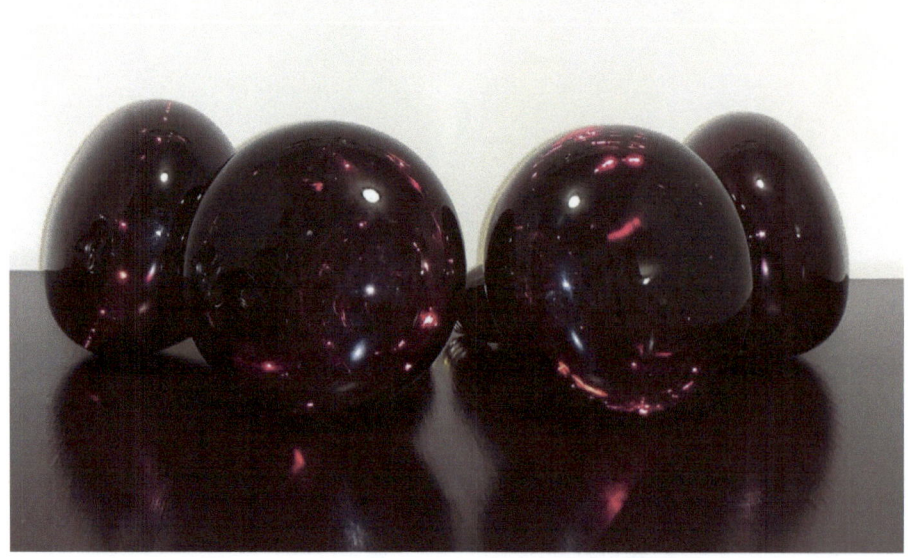

Incandescent infrared bulbs have been in use for more than 50 years. They use the very same technology as the first lightbulb patented by Thomas Edison. Red and other visible light, near infrared energy, and heat are produced by electricity passing through a filament. In order to produce enough of these energies, the bulbs are higher wattage than typical household light bulbs, ranging from 150W to 300W. The bulbs are typically red in color, which reduces the amount of non-red visible light that passes through the bulb in order to keep it from being blindingly bright. The original use for incandescent infrared bulbs was as a heat source, and it is easy to see why. These bulbs get very hot, reaching nearly 600° Fahrenheit in some of the higher wattage versions.

Incandescent infrared bulbs are designed to fit into a standard (size E26/E27) lamp socket, which adds to their convenience and versatility. No special equipment is required to operate them; any lamp with a wattage rating that matches or exceeds that of the bulb will do.

Infrared LEDs

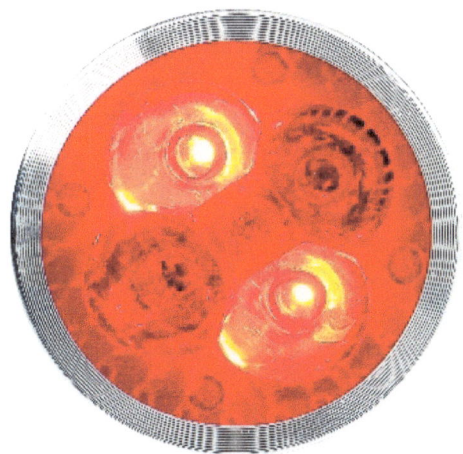

Infrared LEDs are a more recent addition to the infrared light device market. While light-emitting diode (LED) technology has been in use for several decades, LED devices that emit red light and near infrared energy have been widely available to consumers for just over a decade. LED bulbs contain multiple diodes that are programmed to emit energy at specific wavelengths. Unlike incandescent bulbs, LED bulbs produce almost no heat, remaining cool to the touch even after hours of use. They also do not produce "waste light," which is visible light other than red light.

LED bulbs are designed with an E26/E27 screw that allows them to be used in a regular household lamp. Because their wattage is typically low (25W and under) users are able to operate them in lamps they already own. Additionally, LED bulbs are small in size, which allows for multiple bulbs to be used at once to concentrate energy on a specific area.

Factors to Consider When Selecting Infrared Bulbs

How do consumers decide which type and brand of infrared bulb is right for them? Each type of bulb offers some advantages that the other does not. In the sections to follow we'll take a look at factors to consider when deciding on a technology type and comparing brands of bulbs.

Independent Laboratory Testing

When comparing brands of bulbs, you will want to find out if the bulb has been tested in an independent laboratory for two reasons. The first of these is to ensure that the bulbs have been verified to emit near infrared energy, which is not part of the visible light

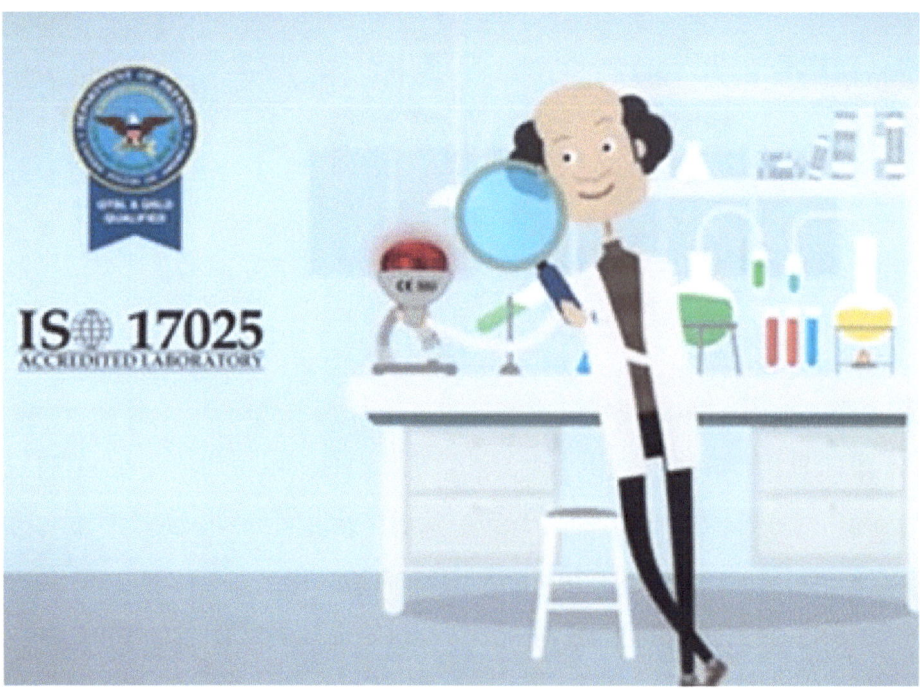

spectrum and, therefore, cannot be seen by the naked eye. Without a lab test, there is no way of verifying that the bulbs emit any infrared energy at all, much less the amount they release. Secondly, data from lab tests allows you to make an apples to apples comparison of the bulb's performance because they were tested using the same methods and equipment as the other manufacturer's bulbs.

Heat

Heat production, or the lack thereof, is one of the biggest differences between incandescent and LED bulbs. If you are purchasing bulbs for use in a home sauna, you will want to choose an incandescent bulb, which can reach nearly 600° Fahrenheit when it reaches peak temperature.

If you are not outfitting a home sauna or not looking to apply heat, an LED bulb is a better choice. LED bulbs can also be added to a sauna or used with an incandescent bulb to increase the amount of red light/NIR energy without producing more heat.

Wavelength Output Distribution

This term refers to the energy emitted at a given wavelength as a percentage of the total output. What you want to look for is a bulb that offers a significant amount of its output in the red light (650nm-699nm) and near infrared (700nm-1000nm) range, with a

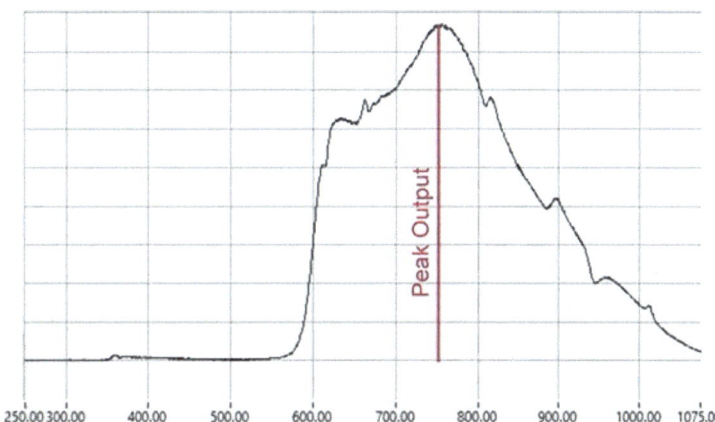

peak wavelength of at least 10% in the NIR range. Output distribution data is offered as either a table of values, a bell curve (histogram), or both.

Irradiance

In addition to the percentage of output within the red and NIR ranges, you want to consider irradiance. This is the amount of energy (of any kind) that the bulb puts out at a given distance. The higher the irradiance number, the more total output of energy.

If this is confusing, you can think of it in terms of a pie. In this analogy, irradiance = the weight of the pie. If you have multiple pies of different weights, then 15% of the heaviest pie will be a larger amount than 15% of the lightest pie.

Non-Toxicity

If you have taken the time to read this book, your health is clearly important to you. Therefore, when considering a red/NIR bulb, you will want to avoid those that contain toxic substances. This is especially true for incandescent bulbs, which are sometimes coated with Teflon to make them resistant to shattering. Bulbs that bear a certification of compliance with the European Union Restriction of Hazardous Substances Directive 2002/95/EC (RoHS) are verified free of multiple toxic substances, including lead, mercury, and Teflon.

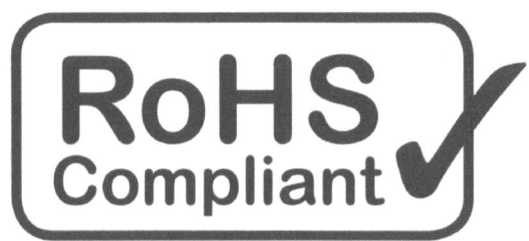

EMF

Electric and magnetic fields (EMFs) are defined by the National Institutes of Health as "invisible areas of energy, often referred to as radiation, that are associated with the use of electrical power and various forms of natural and man-made lighting."

Some consumers wish to avoid devices that produce large amounts of EMF. Fortunately for them, incandescent bulbs, because of the way that they are designed, produce no EMF. It should be noted; however, that if you are looking to minimize or avoid EMF exposure, you will want to consider the EMF output of both the bulb and the lamp being used to operate it.

Read More About . . .

EMF https://www.niehs.nih.gov/health/topics/agents/emf/index.cfm

How to Make a Comparison Among Bulb Brands

Below, we provide a worksheet that you can use to compare infrared products across ten key criteria.

Enter Product Names at Right					
Maximum Operating Temperature					
Time to Reach Maximum Temperature					
Output Range (nm)					
Peak Output Wavelength (nm)					
Power Output in Visible (380nm – 699nm) and Near Infrared (700nm-1000nm) Wavelengths					
Irradiance at 12 inches (.33M)					
Irradiance at 24 inches (.67M)					
Irradiance at 36 inches (1M)					
Fits Standard E26/E27 Socket					
CE Mark					
RoHS Certification					
EMF Output					

Chapter Five: Infrared Light Therapy at Home

One of the most appealing factors of infrared light therapy is that it can easily be conducted at home and with minimal costs. In this section, we're going to discuss the best ways to safely get results from home infrared light therapy.

Building Your Own Infrared Sauna

Infrared saunas are a relaxing way to break a sweat and enjoy the therapeutic potential of infrared light. Because of the safe way infrared lamps produce heat, infrared sauna sessions are less likely to cause faintness or shortness of breath. Users typically report a more comfortable experience from start to finish, and infrared lights help to bestow the fresh, glowing look that we all want.

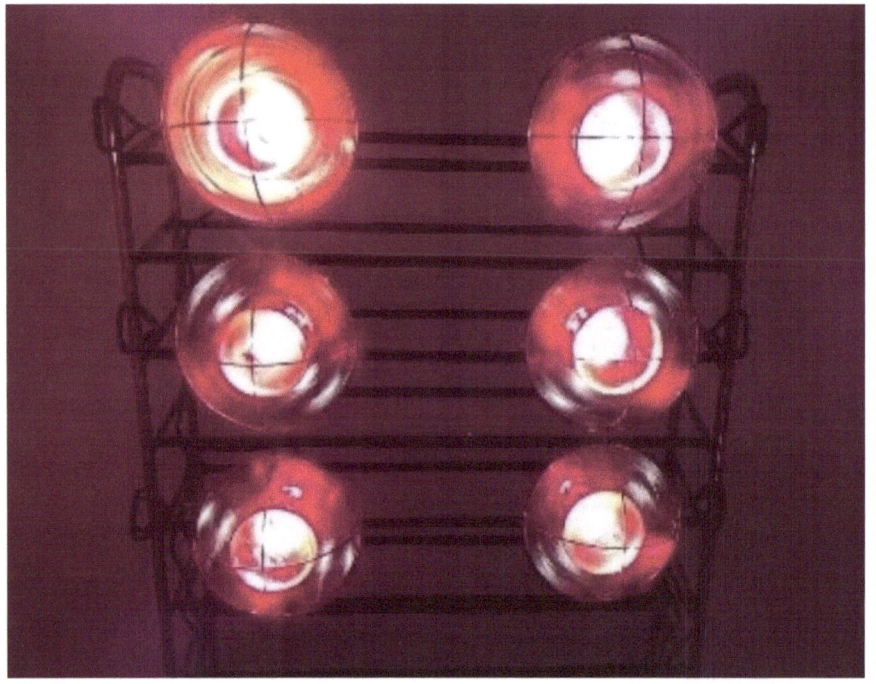

You may have experienced an infrared sauna at a high-end spa -- or even as part of a prescribed medical regimen -- but there are other ways. In fact, many people are building infrared saunas in their own homes, allowing them to relax and rejuvenate whenever they feel the urge!

What About Portable Infrared Saunas?

There are a number of "portable" options available to consumers, many of which look like large canvas tents. While these can be effective, multiple consumers have found that building their own infrared sauna was easier, less expensive, and yielded better results than any of the other options on the market. Now, we're going to show you how you can build your own sauna so you can see for yourself how easy it is.

Getting Started: Understanding How Your Infrared Sauna Will Work

Before we get into the setup of a home sauna, let's take a look at how an infrared sauna actually functions.

First of all, we must consider the heat source. The "heaters" in an infrared sauna don't just heat the air. Your infrared sauna will use a series of bulbs which emit infrared and red light that penetrates your body and warms it. Much of the therapeutic benefit of NIR bulbs comes from the deep, penetrating nature of the light which is able to reach all the way down to deep tissue, even bone.

This is quite different from saunas that use ceramic heaters or hot rocks to produce ambient heat which must be absorbed into the body.

The good news about infrared light is that it's convenient and easy to work with. When it comes to making an infrared sauna at home, you don't need to worry about extremely high levels of humidity, installing high-voltage heaters with GFCI circuits, assembling cedar paneling, or performing any other tasks that might require a contractor.

Step One: Choosing a Location

The first step to creating your own relaxing hideaway at home is to choose where you want it to be. You can use nearly any space to start with. For a semi-permanent installation, you might want to use an extra bathroom, walk-in closet, or other smaller space with low traffic.

Does your area have four walls? A door? A high ceiling? These are factors to consider (we'll talk about why in a moment).

(NOTE: Don't have much space? Many people use their main bathroom for a sauna and simply move their infrared lights out of the way when not in use. This method works, but requires a bit more set up each time you want to use your infrared sauna.)

How Much Space Do You Need?

Typically, the smaller the space, the faster you will heat up. Any small room (around 5' x 5') where you can install a rack of lights on the wall (and possibly the ceiling) can be turned into an infrared sauna. This is why closets are often used.

If you're handy with tools, you can also build an enclosure specifically for your sauna. This isn't necessary, though. The key point is that the sauna will be more effective the smaller it is. You will want to position yourself relatively close (12-18 inches) to the infrared bulbs to experience the full benefits, so turning a spacious living room into a sauna may not be the best idea!

Step Two: Setting Up the Infrared Therapy Lamps

This is where you can get creative. You will need some type of lamp for each of the infrared bulbs, and you will need to make sure that you're setting everything up safely. Watch where you're placing cords to minimize tripping or electrical hazards.

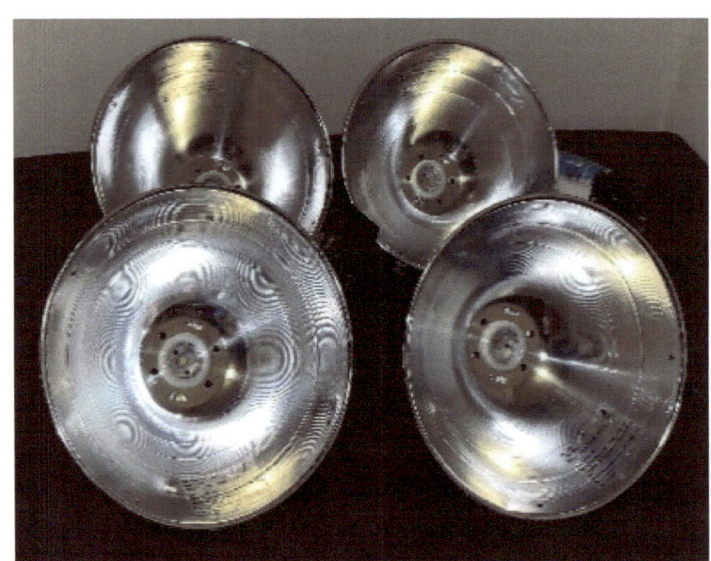

The easiest type of lamp to use for this project is a simple clamp lamp. Make sure you use lamps that are rated for wattage that is equal to or greater than wattage of the bulbs you will be putting into them. You will also want to choose a lamp that has a ceramic socket and metal reflector, which will allow them to withstand the heat produced by the bulbs. For example, you can use Woods Clamp Lights, available on Amazon. Similar lamps are available at most home improvement stores as well.

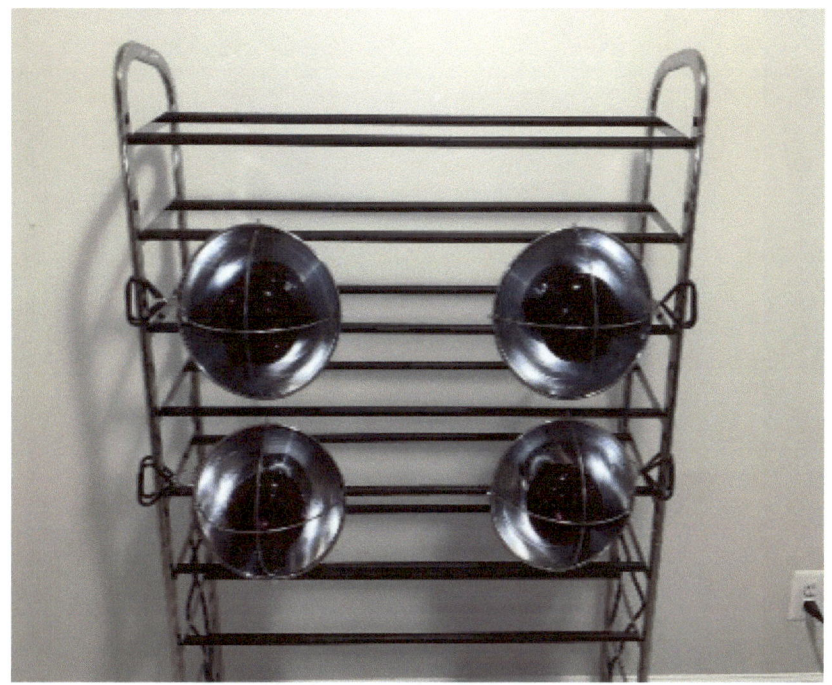

You're also you're going to need something to clamp the lamps to. If your DIY sauna room has a shelf, you're already halfway finished. You can simply attach your array of infrared clamp lamps to the shelves and position them to direct their light output toward you. If you don't have a shelf already in place, a shoe rack will do nicely. You'll want something with two or three different shelves that you can attach lamps to make it easier to obtain full-body coverage. When positioning your infrared therapy lamps, make sure the lamp hoods stay clear of your skin and anything flammable, as they will get hot.

Once you have the lamps mounted, direct the cords out of the way and plug them into a power strip with surge protector. This will not only offer additional electrical safety, but allow you to switch the lamps on and off from a central location. Once this is all in place and your cords are safely out of the way, you're all set. Just grab a thermometer, put on your eye protection, and turn on the bulbs. Monitor the temperature in the sauna and begin your session when the thermometer reads 100° Fahrenheit. Depending on the size of your sauna space and the number of bulbs used, the temperature will most likely continue to rise. Most incandescent infrared bulbs reach maximum operating temperature within 20 minutes. Do not allow the temperature to exceed 120°. If it does reach this temperature, stop your session and open a door or window or turn off one or more of the bulbs.

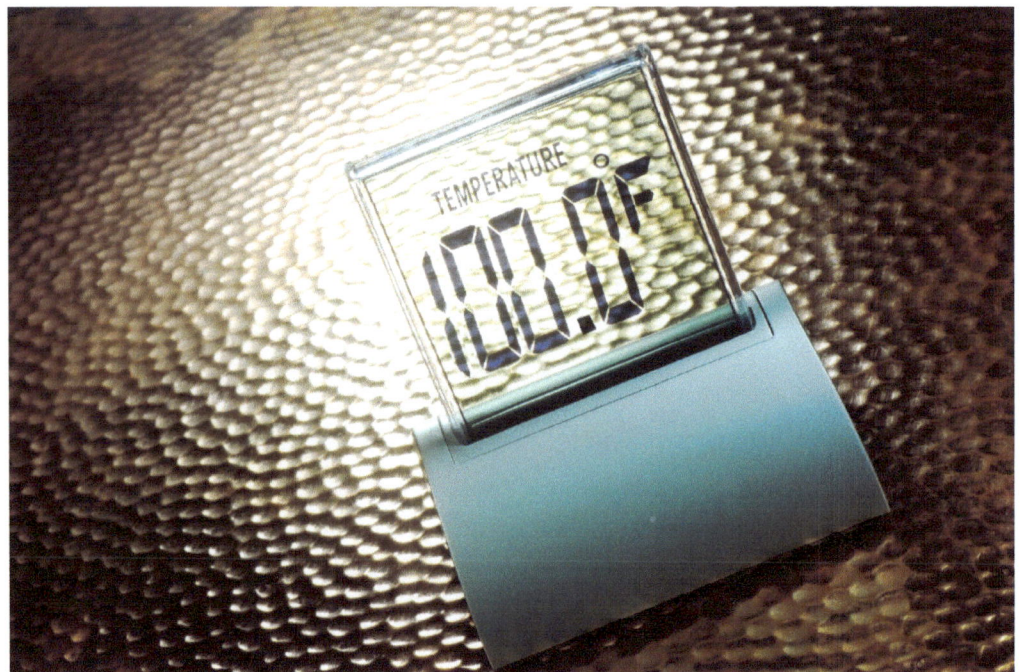

The greatest benefits of infrared therapy come from directed light rather than ambient heat. Point your infrared lamps directly at your body and maintain a distance of 12-18 inches from the bulbs. Avoid pointing the lamps at your head as this can cause rapid overheating. If the warming sensation becomes uncomfortable, move away from the lamps until you feel a relaxing level of heat.

Safe Use of Your Home Infrared Sauna

When using your sauna, it's important to follow some basic safety guidelines. Here are some things to keep in mind:

- Check with your doctor before using any type of sauna.

- Do not look directly into the infrared lamps. Just like any bright light, they can damage your eyes over time. Use protective eyewear whenever you're in your sauna.

- If you've set up your sauna in a bathroom or near water, be sure to use a power strip with a ground-fault circuit and plug your lamps into a GFCI outlet. Be cautious of any potential electrical hazards.

- If your sauna makes you sweat heavily, be sure to supplement fluids and electrolytes before and after your sessions. Hydration is important, but so is replacing lost minerals and salts.

Getting the Best Quality Infrared Sauna Bulbs

Your overall results from this project will depend on a few factors. Not only will the size of your selected sauna space play a role, but so will the quality and output of your near infrared bulbs.

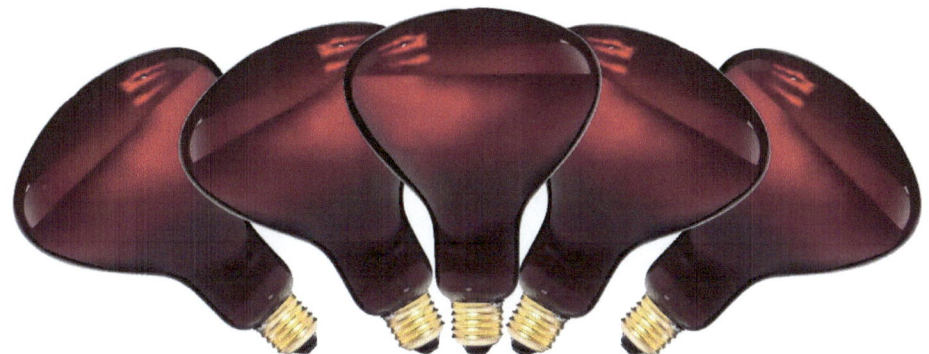

Not all infrared therapy bulbs are the same. Differences in manufacturing processes, materials, and quality control have a huge impact on your results. In order to be an infrared bulb, it must emit energy in the infrared range of 700nm-3000nm. Most bulbs marketed for consumer use produce near infrared, which is the shorter-wavelength portion of the infrared spectrum, ranging from 700nm-1000nm.

You'll want a bulb that is produced without hazardous substances such as heavy metals or Teflon, which can produce hazardous fumes at high temperatures. A good way to ensure that the bulbs are free of these substances is to look for an RoHS certification, which is an assurance that the bulb is free from lead, mercury, Teflon, and other substances identified in the European Union Restriction of Hazardous Substances Directive 2002/95/EC. For additional guidance on selecting bulbs, refer to Chapter Five.

Chapter Six: Infrared Light Therapy Safety

Light therapy is generally safe and research has revealed few dangers or risks with regular use. That being said, it's important to review safety precautions and contraindications, even if there are few.

First and foremost, **consult a medical professional before beginning NIR/red light therapy.**

Second, you will be using an electric lamp to operate a glass lightbulb that reaches temperatures in excess of 500 degrees. There are some basic safety precautions to keep in mind:

1. Wear eye protection while using the bulb. Avoid looking directly at the bulb while it is lit.
2. Maintain a distance of at least 12 inches from the bulb when in operation
3. Keep anything that is flammable or can be damaged by heat at least 12 inches from the bulb. This includes but is not limited to clothing, carpets, paper, wood, and plastic.
4. Do not leave the bulb unattended while in use. Do not fall asleep while using the bulb.
5. Do not use near water or immerse the bulb in water.
6. Do not touch the bulb immediately after use. Let it cool down first.
7. Do not touch the bulb if you have oil or lotion on your hands.
8. Be cautious when handling glass bulbs as they can shatter if dropped or struck.
9. Make sure that the lamp you use to operate your NIR bulb is designed to operate bulbs that have the same or greater wattage. You can usually find this information on the side of the socket or on the cord.

Lastly, one of the only dangers posed by NIR/red light (or any heat source) is overheating. Do not exceed the time limit recommended by your medical professional. If you feel yourself overheating, move away from or turn off the bulb.

Chapter Seven: Infrared Light Therapy FAQ

Q: Can I wear makeup when using infrared therapy on my face?

A: Makeup does not affect the therapeutic effects of the light.

Q: Can I wear my clothes between my skin and the therapy light?

A: Near infrared / red light energy is capable of penetrating clothing, so you may keep your clothes on if you prefer. Because of the heat produced by the bulb, you may prefer to wear lighter clothing, especially if you are in a sauna.

Q: Will NIR therapy interact with any medications I use?

A: While drug interactions are rare, consult a medical professional before beginning therapy.

Q: Will Infrared light help with Seasonal Affective Disorder (SAD)?

A: Studies have shown that red light and NIR, as well as other light therapies, can improve the symptoms of Seasonal Affective Disorder (SAD).

Q: How warm does the treatment site get? Does NIR therapy burn?

A: At a proper distance, red light/NIR therapy feel like compared to direct sunlight on a warm, cloudless day. If you feel uncomfortably warm, move further away from the bulb or end the session.

Q: Do I need to wear some sort of eye protection like when using a tanning bed?

A: Eye protection is strongly recommended. Options range from tanning goggles to glasses designed specifically for use with NIR and red light. Even while wearing eye protection, avoid directing red, IR, and NIR light directly into the eye.

Glossary

Adenosine Triphosphate (ATP): A molecule that carries energies within a cell; often referred to as a cell's "power plant".

Anti-Oxidant: A substance that removes potentially damaging oxidizing substances from a living organism

Bioactive Light: Forms of light that have some sort of measurable effect on the human body. These include UV light, Infrared light, and blue light.

Blue Light: Blue light is a color in the light spectrum that's visible to the naked eye. Because blue light is a short wavelength it produces higher amounts of energy and thus can cause headaches and eye strain.

Cellular Respiration: The process carried out by cells to convert fuel to energy and nutrients.

Electromagnetic Spectrum: The range of radiation that encompasses gamma rays, x-rays, microwaves, and radio signals as well as visible and near infrared light.

Endorphins: Chemicals produced by the pituitary gland and central nervous system that help the body manage stress and regulate responses to pain.

Far Infrared (NIR) Light: The longest wavelengths of infrared light, comprising the wavelengths of 1001nm-3000nm.

Free Radical: Oxygen molecules with uneven numbers of electrons. This uneven number causes these molecules to seek out other molecules and bind to them, which can often result in reactions that are harmful to the body.

Incandescent Lightbulb: A bulb that produces light and heat as a result of electrical current passing through a metal filament.

Infrared Light: That portion of the electromagnetic spectrum that includes the long wavelength, or red, end of the visible-light range and into the microwave range. Infrared light is invisible to the naked eye but can be felt as warmth on the skin.

Visible Light: The portion of the electromagnetic spectrum that is visible to the human eye. In discussions of bioactive light, this spectrum may include invisible or nearly-visible light as well.

Nanometer: The unit of measure used to describe the wavelengths of the types of energy in the electromagnetic spectrum.

Near Infrared (NIR) Light: The shortest wavelengths of infrared light, comprising the wavelengths of 700nm-1000nm.

Nitric Oxide: A chemical that is comprised of a nitrogen atom and an oxygen atom. It performs a number of functions in the body relative to cellular function

Photobiomodulation: Using red and near infrared light to trigger chemical changes within cells.

Photons: Particles of light

Red Light: Visible light with wavelengths between 650nm-699nm.

Thermotherapy: The process of treating the body using high or low temperatures.

Ultraviolet (UV) Light: Ultraviolet (UV) light falls in the range of the EM spectrum between visible light and X-rays, having wavelengths from 10nm-379nm.

Vasodilation: Enlargement of the blood vessels.

Wavelength: A way of categorizing energy on the electromagnetic spectrum. The wavelength is the amount of time between the highest and lowest points on the wave of energy.

White Light: Visible light

www.ingramcontent.com/pod-product-compliance
Lightning Source LLC
Chambersburg PA
CBHW051218220526
45473CB00003B/1077